Copyright 2023

All right reserved. No part of this book should be reproduced without express permission of the author.

Reproduction of all or any part of this book is punishable under relevant law.

Table of Contents

Osteoporosis causes bones to become weak and brittle — so brittle that a fall or even mild stresses such as bending over or coughing can cause a fracture. Osteoporosis-related fractures most commonly occur in the hip, wrist or spine.

Bone is living tissue that is constantly being broken down and replaced. Osteoporosis occurs when the creation of new bone doesn't keep up with the loss of old bone.

Osteoporosis affects men and women of all races. But white and Asian women, especially older women who are past menopause, are at highest risk. Medications, healthy diet and weight-bearing exercise can help prevent bone loss or strengthen already weak bones.

BREAKFAST

1. Tater Tot Breakfast Casserole

Prep Time: 1hrs 30 Minutes

Cook Time: 2hrs 55 Minutes

Servings: 8

Ingredients

- One 16-ounce bag frozen Tater Tots
- Butter, for the baking dish
- 1 tablespoon olive oil
- 1 pound spicy bulk breakfast sausage
- 1 medium onion, very finely diced
- 1 cup milk
- 1/2 cup half-and-half
- 1/4 teaspoon seasoned salt
- 1/4 teaspoon cayenne
- 4 large eggs
- 1 red bell pepper, very finely diced
- 1 green bell pepper, very finely diced

- 2 cups grated Cheddar cheese
- 1 cup grated pepper jack cheese
- Salt and freshly ground black pepper

Instructions

1. Line up the tater tots in a buttered 9-by-13-inch baking dish.

2. Add the olive oil to a large skillet over medium heat. Add the sausage and onion and cook, breaking the sausage up with a wooden spoon, until browned and cooked through, 8 to 10 minutes. Set aside to cool slightly, then sprinkle it over the tater tots.

3. In a large bowl, mix the milk, half-and-half, seasoned salt, cayenne, eggs, bell peppers, half of both cheeses and some salt and pepper. Pour over the tots and sausage mixture, then top with the rest of the cheese. Cover with foil and refrigerate overnight.

4. Preheat the oven to 350 degrees F.

5. Bake, covered, for about 25 minutes. Remove the foil and continue to bake until the cheese is brown and bubbly and the casserole is cooked through, another 20 to 35 minutes. Cut into squares and serve.

Prep Time: 30 Minutes

Cook Time: 1hrs 55 Minutes

Servings: 8-10

Ingredients

- 2 1/2 cups frozen potato tots
- One 12-ounce package pork breakfast sausage
- 10 strips bacon (8 ounces)
- 5 large eggs
- 2 cups grated American cheese (6 ounces)
- 2 cups grated white Cheddar (6 ounces)
- All-purpose flour, for dusting 1 1/2 pounds store-bought pizza dough (see Cook's Note)
- Ketchup and/or hot sauce, for serving

Instructions

1. Preheat the oven to 425 degrees F. Line a baking sheet with parchment and spread the potato tots on the sheet. Bake until golden brown and crisp, about 25

minutes. Transfer the baking sheet to a wire rack and let cool. Lower the oven to 400 degrees F.

2. Meanwhile, heat the sausage in a large nonstick skillet over medium heat and cook, stirring to break up the sausage, until browned and no longer pink, about 8 minutes. Transfer the sausage to paper towels with a slotted spoon to drain; discard any remaining fat. Let the sausage cool, then crumble into 1/2-inch pieces.

3. Heat the bacon in the skillet over medium heat and cook, flipping once, until browned, about 8 minutes. Using tongs, transfer the bacon to paper towels to drain; discard any remaining fat. Let the bacon cool, then crumble into 1/2-inch pieces.

4. Prepare a bowl of ice water and set aside. Cover 4 eggs by 1 inch with water in a small saucepan and bring to a boil. Cover the pan, remove from the heat and let the eggs stand for 6 minutes. Uncover and drain the eggs, then transfer to the bowl of ice water and let stand for 3 minutes. Drain and peel the eggs, then quarter each egg lengthwise.

5. Toss the American cheese and Cheddar together in a small bowl until evenly combined.

6. Roll the dough into a 20-by-14-inch rectangle on a lightly floured work surface. Starting from the shorter

end, spread the cheese mixture evenly over half of the dough, leaving a 1-inch border on the sides. Scatter the sausage, bacon and potato tots evenly over the cheese. Arrange all the egg quarters, yolk up, along the short side of the rectangle. Working from this short side, tightly roll the dough up, jelly roll-style, into a log. Pinch the open seams together to seal, then tuck them underneath the log.

7. Beat the remaining egg. Transfer the log to the prepared baking sheet and brush with the egg wash. Bake until the bread is golden brown all over, about 40 minutes.

8. Let the bread cool for 10 minutes. Halve the bread lengthwise, cut each half crosswise into 4 equal pieces and serve warm with ketchup or hot sauce.

Prep Time: 25 Minutes

Cook Time:55 Minutes

Servings: 12

Ingredients

- 1 pound breakfast sausage, hot or mild
- 1/3 cup all-purpose flour
- 3 to 4 cups whole milk, more to taste
- 1/2 teaspoon seasoned salt
- 2 teaspoons freshly ground black pepper, more to taste
- Biscuits, warmed, for serving

Instructions

1. With your finger, tear small pieces of sausage and add them in a single layer to a large heavy skillet. Brown the sausage over medium-high heat until no longer pink. Reduce the heat to medium-low. Sprinkle on half the flour and stir so that the sausage soaks it all up, then add more little by little. Stir it around and

cook it for another minute or so, then pour in the milk, stirring constantly.

2. Cook the gravy, stirring frequently, until it thickens. (This may take a good 10 to 12 minutes.) Sprinkle in the seasoned salt and pepper and continue cooking until very thick and luscious. If it gets too thick too soon, just splash in another 1/2 cup of milk or more if needed. Taste and adjust the seasoning.

3. Spoon the sausage gravy over warm biscuits and serve immediately!

Prep Time: 25 Minutes

Cook Time: 35 Minutes

Servings: 8-10

Ingredients

For the salsa:

- 1 14-ounce can whole tomatoes
- 1 10-ounce can diced tomatoes and green chiles
- 1 10-ounce can diced tomatoes and green chiles
- 1/4 cup fresh cilantro (or more to taste)
- 2 tablespoons chopped onion
- 1 small clove garlic, minced
- 1/2 jalapeno pepper, thinly sliced
- 1/4 teaspoon sugar
- 1/4 teaspoon ground cumin
- Salt
- Juice of 1/2 lime

For the pizza:

- 1 pound thick-cut peppered bacon

- 2 tablespoons vegetable oil, plus more for the baking sheet
- 2 cups frozen hash browns
- 1 red bell pepper, chopped
- 1 green bell pepper, chopped
- 1 pound store-bought pizza dough, thawed if frozen
- 12 ounces fresh mozzarella, sliced
- 8 large eggs
- Salt and freshly ground pepper

Instructions

1. Make the salsa: Combine the whole tomatoes with their juices, diced tomatoes, cilantro, onion, garlic, jalapeno, sugar, cumin, 1/4 teaspoon salt and the lime juice in a food processor or blender. Pulse several times until it reaches the consistency you like. Set aside.

2. Prepare the pizza: Place the oven rack in the lowest position and preheat to 475 degrees F. Fry the bacon in a large skillet over medium heat, turning occasionally, until chewy, about 8 minutes; drain on paper towels. Chop into bite-size pieces.

3. Meanwhile, heat 1 tablespoon vegetable oil in a separate large skillet over medium-high heat; add the frozen hash browns and cook, stirring occasionally, until they just start turning golden brown, about 7 minutes. Remove from the pan and set aside. In the same skillet, fry the red and green peppers in the remaining 1 tablespoon vegetable oil over

4. medium-high heat until they're nice and brown, about 5 minutes. Set aside.

5. Roll out the pizza dough on a lightly oiled baking sheet. Spread 1/2 cup salsa over the dough, then evenly distribute the sliced mozzarella over the salsa. Sprinkle with the hash browns, bell peppers and bacon.

6. Next comes the fun part! Make 8 little wells in the filling here and there all over the surface of the pizza; crack the eggs into the wells. Sprinkle with salt and pepper to taste. Bake until the crust is golden brown and the eggs are set but still slightly soft, about 15 minutes. Cut into large pieces and serve with the remaining salsa.

Prep Time: 15 Minutes

Cook Time: 40 Minutes

Servings: 12

Ingredients

- Butter, for greasing the pan
- 2 tablespoons extra-virgin olive oil
- Two 3-to-4-ounce sweet or spicy Italian sausage links, casings removed
- 2 cloves garlic, minced
- 1 cup shredded smoked mozzarella (4 ounces)
- 4 large eggs, at room temperature
- 2 cups milk, at room temperature
- 1 1/2 cups all-purpose flour
- 2 small green onions, pale green and white parts only, finely sliced to yield 1/4 cup
- 3 tablespoons chopped fresh basil
- 1 1/2 teaspoons salt
- 1/2 teaspoon freshly ground black pepper
- Maple syrup, for drizzling

Instructions

1. Special equipment: One 12-cup nonstick muffin pan, each cup about 1/2-cup capacity, or a 12-cup popover pan, each cup about 1/2-cup capacity

2. Place an oven rack in the center of the oven and preheat to 400 degrees F. Butter the muffin cups.

3. Heat the oil over medium heat in a medium nonstick skillet. Add the sausage and break it into 1/4-to-1/2-inch pieces using a wooden spoon. Cook until brown and cooked through, about 6 minutes. Add the garlic and cook until aromatic, about 30 seconds. Spoon about 1 1/2 tablespoons sausage into each muffin cup. Sprinkle the cheese on top of the sausage.

4. Blend the eggs in a blender until frothy, about 15 seconds. Add the milk, flour, green onions, basil, salt and pepper. Blend until just incorporated. Pour the batter into the muffin cups, filling each cup to just below the rim. Bake, without opening the oven door, until puffed and golden, about 35 minutes.

5. Place the popovers on a platter and drizzle with maple syrup.

Prep Time: 15 Minutes

Cook Time: 1hrs 40 Minutes

Servings: 12

Ingredients

Butter, for greasing

- 1/2 loaf of sliced white loaf bread
- 1 pound fresh bulk pork sausage with sage
- 10 ounces sharp Cheddar, grated
- 2 cups half-and-half
- 1 teaspoon dry mustard
- 1 teaspoon salt
- 5 large eggs, lightly beaten

Instructions

1. Cut the bread into 1-inch cubes and spread in the bottom of a greased 9- by 13- by 2- inch casserole dish.

2. In a medium skillet, brown the sausage over medium heat until fully cooked and no longer pink. Remove the sausage with a slotted spoon to drain the fat. Spread the cooked sausage over the bread and top with the cheese. Then stir together the, half-and-half, dry mustard, salt and eggs. Pour this mixture over the cheese. Cover the casserole with aluminum foil and refrigerate for 8 hours or overnight.

3. The next day, preheat the oven to 350 degrees F.

4. Bake the covered casserole until set and slightly golden, about 50 minutes. Remove from the oven and allow the casserole to set for 15 minutes before serving.

Prep Time: 55 Minutes

Cook Time: 1hrs 40 Minutes

Servings: 8

Ingredients

- 2 pounds sage sausage
- 2 Granny Smith apples, diced
- 1 large yellow onion, diced
- 1 tablespoon chopped fresh sage
- 12 large eggs
- 2 cups whole milk
- 1/2 cup half-and-half
- salt and freshly ground black pepper
- Salted butter, for greasing the lasagna pan
- 6 cinnamon raisin English muffins, cut into bite-size chunks
- 2 1/2 cups grated white Cheddar
- 2 tablespoons chopped fresh parsley

Instructions

1. Set a large skillet over medium heat and add the sausage. Cook until browned and cooked through, 7 to 9 minutes. Remove the sausage with a slotted spoon and drain on a paper towel lined plate. Without cleaning the skillet, add the apples, onion and sage and cook until the onion has softened, 2 to 3 minutes. Remove the pan from the heat and set aside.

2. Mix together the eggs, milk and half-and-half in a large pitcher or bowl. Season with salt and pepper and set aside.

3. Grease a large casserole dish with some butter. Layer in half the English muffins, half the sausage, half the apple/onion mixture and half the cheese. Repeat with the other half of the same ingredients, ending with the cheese. Slowly pour the egg mixture all over the top. Cover with plastic wrap and refrigerate overnight.

4. Remove the pan from the fridge 20 to 30 minutes before baking. Preheat the oven to 350 degrees F.

5. Replace the plastic wrap on top of the casserole with aluminum foil. Bake for 35 to 40 minutes, then remove the foil and continue to bake until the top is golden brown and slightly crisp, 10 to 15 minutes more.

6. Sprinkle with the chopped parsley. Serve warm and enjoy.

Prep Time: 10 Minutes

Cook Time: 40 Minutes

Ingredients

- 2 cups milk
- 2 large eggs
- 4 tablespoons unsalted butter, melted and cooled, plus more for brushing
- 1/2 teaspoon pure vanilla extract
- 1 1/4 cups all-purpose flour
- 3 tablespoons sugar
- 1/4 teaspoon salt
- Butter and maple syrup or jam, for serving

Instructions

1. Whisk the milk, eggs, melted butter and vanilla in a large bowl until combined. Add the flour, sugar and salt; whisk until the batter is smooth, with no lumps.

2. Heat a medium nonstick skillet over medium heat; lightly brush with butter. Add 1/4 cup batter; swirl the skillet to coat the bottom with a thin layer of the batter. Cook until set on top and lightly browned around the edge, about 1 1/2 minutes. Gently lift and flip the pancake with a rubber spatula; cook until just browned on the other side, about 15 more seconds. Transfer to a plate and repeat with the remaining batter (do not brush the skillet with more butter). Fold into quarters and serve with butter and syrup or jam.

Prep Time: 35 Minutes

Cook Time: 15 Minutes

Servings: 6

Ingredients

- Nonstick cooking spray, for the pan, optional
- Salted butter, at room temperature, for the pan and/or spreading, optional10 large eggs
- 1/2 cup whole milk
- salt and freshly ground black pepper
- Extra-virgin olive oil
- 8 ounces cremini mushrooms, sliced
- 3 cups stemmed spinach
- 6 slices Swiss cheese (about 6 ounces)
- 6 English muffins, split

Instructions

1. Preheat the oven to 375 degrees. Spray a 9-by-13-inch baking pan with nonstick cooking spray or grease with butter.

2. Heat 1 tablespoon of the olive oil over medium-high heat. Add the mushrooms and cook, stirring occasionally, until wilted and beginning to brown; about 5 minutes. Add the spinach, 1 teaspoon salt and a few grinds of pepper. Cook until spinach just begins to wilt, stirring occasionally, about 2 minutes. Remove pan from heat and set aside to cool.

3. Whisk the eggs, milk, 1 teaspoon salt and a few grinds of pepper together in a large bowl. Gently whisk in the cooled mushroom mixture, then pour the egg mixture into the prepared pan. Bake until puffed and set, 15 to 20 minutes. Remove from the oven and let cool.

4. Place the English muffins cut-side up on a baking sheet and brush with some butter if using. Bake until slightly toasty, 3 to 4 minutes.

5. Once the eggs are cool enough to handle, use a large round biscuit cutter (about 3 3/4 inches in diameter) or the rim of a juice glass to cut out 6 rounds of egg. (For ways to use the leftover egg scraps,.) Using an offset spatula or a butter knife, remove each egg round from the pan and place on bottom half of an English muffin. Top each with a slice of Swiss cheese and the other muffin half. Wrap each sandwich individually with aluminum foil, put in a resealable

plastic bag and freeze up to 1 month or refrigerate for up to 1 week.

6. To reheat, unwrap a sandwich and place on a paper towel on a microwave-safe dish. Microwave 1 to 1 1/2 minutes, until the cheese is melted and eggs are warmed through. Alternatively, thaw a foil-wrapped frozen sandwich overnight in the refrigerator, then bake in a 425-degree F oven until warmed through and the cheese is melted, about 10 minutes.

Prep Time: 35 Minutes

Cook Time: 15 Minutes

Servings: 6

Ingredients

- 2 salmon fillets, sustainably sourced or organic
- 10 to 12 Brussels sprouts, chopped in half
- 1 bunch kale, washed and shredded
- ½ head cauliflower, pulsed into cauliflower rice (you can use a whole cauliflower head if you wish)
- 3 tablespoons olive or coconut oil
- 1 teaspoon curry powder
- salt

For marinade:

- ¼ cup tamari sauce
- 1 teaspoon Dijon mustard
- 1 teaspoon sesame oil
- 1 teaspoon honey or maple syrup (optional)
- 1 tablespoon sesame seeds

Instructions

1. Preheat oven to 350°F.

2. Line a baking tray and add chopped Brussels sprouts. Coat with 1 tablespoon oil and season with salt. Add to oven and roast for 20 minutes.

3. Meanwhile, make marinade by combining all ingredients in a bowl and whisking until combined.

4. Remove Brussels sprouts after 20 minutes and add salmon fillets to the baking tray. Spoon marinade over salmon fillets and return to oven for a further 13 to 15 minutes, or until salmon is cooked to your liking.

5. While salmon is cooking, heat a pan over medium-high heat and add 1 tablespoon oil. Add kale and sauté until wilted (2 to 3 minutes). Remove from pan and set aside.

6. Heat remaining oil in pan and add cauliflower rice. Season with 1 teaspoon curry powder and salt and sauté until cooked (2 to 3 minutes).

7. Remove salmon and Brussels sprouts from oven and divide into two bowls. Add sautéed kale and cauliflower rice to bowls.

11. Best Stuffed Shells

Prep Time: 30 Minutes

Cook Time: 35 Minutes

Servings: 8

Ingredients

- 1 pound (16 ounces) fresh baby spinach or baby kale, or frozen spinach or kale, or 1 ½ pounds Tuscan kale or spinach bunches, washed and stems removed
- 1 tablespoon extra virgin olive oil
- 12 ounces jumbo shells
- 4 cloves garlic, peeled and cut into several segments
- 15 ounces (or 1 pound) ricotta cheese or cottage cheese
- 8 ounces (2 cups) grated part-skim mozzarella, divided
- ½ cup (2 ounces) grated Parmesan, plus extra for garnish
- ¼ cup (⅔-ounce) chives or green onions (mostly green parts), cut into ¼-long pieces

- Freshly ground pepper, to taste
- ½ teaspoon red pepper flakes, to taste (omit if sensitive to spice)
- ¾ teaspoon fine sea salt, to taste
- 1 large egg, lightly beaten with a fork
- 3 cups (24 ounces) marinara sauce, homemade* or store-bought (I used Rao's)
- Fresh basil for garnish, optional

Instructions

1. Preheat the oven to 375 with racks in the middle and upper third of the oven. Bring a large Dutch oven or stockpot of water to boil over high heat. Generously salt the water (use at least 2 teaspoons). If you're not using frozen greens, fill a large bowl with ice water for blanching.

2. If you're using fresh greens, add them to the boiling water and cook just until wilted, about 20 to 40 seconds. Using tongs (leave the water in the pot), transfer the greens to the ice bath and let them cool down. Drain off the water and squeeze as much excess water from the greens as possible. Set aside. (If you're using frozen greens, place them in a colander and run

cool water over them until they've full defrosted. Squeeze out as much excess water as possible, and set aside.)

3. Bring the water in the pot back to a boil. Gently add the pasta shells in handfuls so they don't break on the way in. Cook until pliable but just shy of al dente, about 10 minutes, stirring often so they don't stick to the pot. Drain off the water, return the noodles to the pot, and gently stir in the olive oil to prevent the noodles from sticking. Set aside.

4. Turn on your food processor and drop the garlic through the feeding tube. Once the garlic is chopped and stuck to the sides of the bowl, stop the machine and scrape down the sides. For good measure, squeeze off any remaining water in the greens, then add them to the bowl. Process until the greens are chopped into small pieces.

5. Add the ricotta and process until well blended. Add half of the mozzarella, reserving the rest for topping. Add all of the Parmesan and chives, about 10 twists of black pepper, the red pepper flakes and salt. Blend well. Taste, and add additional salt, pepper or red pepper flakes if desired. Finally, add the egg and process until blended. Set aside.

6. If you have an extra-large baking dish (larger than 9×13 inches), spread 1 cup of the marinara sauce across the bottom. Otherwise, divide 1 cup marinara between a large (9×13 inches) and medium-sized baker (say, an 8-inch square). You might need to add another splash of sauce to evenly coat the bottom of the pans.

7. Stuff each intact shell with a heaping spoonful (about 1 ½ to 2 tablespoons) of the green mixture. Place each stuffed shell in the baker in rows. (You might have a few leftover or broken shells; save them for another use.) Spoon the remaining marinara sauce over the tops of the shells. Top the shells with the remaining mozzarella.

8. Cover the baker(s) tightly with foil and bake on the middle rack for 30 minutes. Then, remove the foil and place the bakers on the upper rack. Bake for 5 to 10 more minutes, until the mozzarella is fully melted and turning just slightly golden (you can bake longer for a more golden effect, but the greens will become less vibrant).

9. Garnish the shells with a light dusting of grated Parmesan and some small or torn fresh basil leaves.

Leftover shells will keep well in the refrigerator for up to 4 days, or freeze them for several months.

Prep Time: 15 Minutes

Cook Time: 35 Minutes

Servings: 2

Ingredients

- 2 tablespoons coconut oil or quality high-heat oil such as avocado oil, divided
- 2 eggs, whisked together with a dash of salt
- 2 big cloves garlic, pressed or minced
- ¾ cup chopped green onions (about 1 bunch)

Optional:

- 1 cup chopped vegetables, like bell pepper, carrot or Brussels sprouts
- 1 medium bunch kale (preferably Lacinato but curly green is good, too), ribs removed and leaves chopped
- ¼ teaspoon fine sea salt
- ¾ cup large, unsweetened coconut flakes (not shredded coconut)
- 2 cups cooked and chilled brown rice
- 2 teaspoons reduced-sodium tamari or soy sauce

- 2 teaspoons chili garlic sauce or sriracha
- 1 lime, halved
- Handful fresh cilantro, for garnish

Instructions

1. Heat a large (12-inch or wider) wok, cast iron skillet or non-stick frying pan over medium-high heat. Once the pan is hot enough that a drop of water sizzles on contact, add 1 teaspoon oil and swirl the pan to coat the bottom. Pour in the eggs and cook, stirring frequently, until the eggs are scrambled and lightly set. Transfer the eggs to your empty bowl. Wipe out the pan if necessary with a paper towel (be careful, it's hot!).

2. Add 1 tablespoon oil to the pan and add the garlic, green onions and optional additional vegetables. Cook until fragrant or until the vegetables are tender, stirring frequently, for 30 seconds or longer. Add the kale and salt. Continue to cook until the kale is wilted and tender, stirring frequently, about 1 to 2 minutes. Transfer the contents of the pan to your bowl of eggs.

3. Add the remaining 2 teaspoons oil to the pan. Pour in the coconut flakes and cook, stirring frequently, until

the flakes are lightly golden, about 30 seconds. Add the rice to the pan and cook, stirring occasionally, until the rice is hot, about 3 minutes.

4. Pour the contents of the bowl back into the pan, breaking up the scrambled egg with your spatula or spoon. Once warmed, remove the pan from the heat.

5. Add the tamari, chili garlic sauce and juice of ½ lime. Stir to combine. Taste, and if it's not fantastic yet, add another teaspoon of tamari or a pinch of salt, as needed.

6. Slice the remaining ½ lime into wedges, then divide the fried rice into individual bowls. Garnish with wedges of lime and a sprinkling of torn cilantro leaves, with jars of tamari, chili garlic sauce and/or red pepper flakes on the side, for those who might want more.

Prep Time: 20 Minutes

Cook Time: 60 Minutes

Servings: 5

Ingredients

Filling:

- 1 ¼ pounds sweet potatoes (2 small-to-medium)
- 1 can (15 ounces) black beans, rinsed and drained, or 1 ½ cups cooked black beans
- 4 ounces (1 cup) grated Monterey Jack cheese
- 2 ounces (½ cup) crumbled feta cheese
- 2 small cans (4 ounces each) diced green chiles
- 1 medium jalapeño, seeded and minced
- 2 cloves garlic, pressed or minced
- 2 tablespoons lime juice
- ½ teaspoon ground cumin
- ½ teaspoon chili powder
- ¼ teaspoon cayenne pepper (optional)
- ¼ teaspoon salt, more to taste
- Freshly ground black pepper

- Remaining Ingredients

- 2 cups (16 ounces) mild salsa verde, either homemade or store-bought

- 10 corn tortillas

- 4 ounces (1 cup) grated Monterey Jack cheese

- 2 tablespoons sour cream

- 1 tablespoon water

- ¼ cup chopped red onion

- ¼ cup chopped fresh cilantro

Instructions

1. Preheat the oven to 400 degrees Fahrenheit and line a large baking sheet with parchment paper for easy cleanup.

2. Slice the sweet potatoes in half lengthwise and coat the flat sides lightly with olive oil. Place the sweet potatoes flat-side down on the baking sheet. Bake until they're tender and cooked through, about 30 to 35 minutes. Leave the oven on, since we'll bake the assembled enchiladas soon (no temperature adjustments necessary).

3. Meanwhile, pour enough salsa verde into a 9 by 13-inch baking dish to lightly cover the bottom (about ½

cup). In a medium mixing bowl, combine all of the remaining filling ingredients.

4. Once the sweet potatoes are cooked through and cool enough to handle, scoop out the insides with a spoon. Discard the potato skins, and lightly mash the sweet potatoes with a fork or the back of a spoon.

5. Stir the mashed sweet potato into the bowl of filling, and season to taste with additional salt (I added ¼ teaspoon) and pepper.

6. Warm up your tortillas, one by one in a skillet, or all at once in a microwave so they don't break when you bend them. Wrap them in a clean tea towel so they stay warm.

7. Working with one tortilla at a time, spread about ½ cup filling down the center each tortilla, then wrap both sides over the filling and place it in your baking dish. Repeat for all of the tortillas.

8. Top with the remaining salsa verde and cheese. Bake for 25 to 35 minutes, until sauce is bubbling and the cheese is lightly golden.

9. Let the enchiladas cool for about 5 minutes. Whisk the sour cream and water together to make a drizzly sour cream sauce. Drizzle it back and forth over the

enchiladas, then top them with cilantro and red onion.
Serve.

Prep Time: 30 Minutes

Cook Time: 90 Minutes

Servings: 4

Ingredients

- ½ batch Black Beans (or make the full batch for leftovers)
- 1 batch Cilantro Lime Brown Rice
- 1 batch Quick-Pickled Onions
- 1 batch Cilantro Hemp Pesto (double if you love sauce)

Optional additions:

- Fried eggs or scrambled eggs, toasted pepitas (green pumpkin seeds), crumbled Cotija or feta cheese, sliced avocado, handful of halved cherry tomatoes, hot sauce or quick collard greens

Instructions

1. Prepare each component according to directions (the beans will take the longest, approximately 1 to 2+ hours on the stove, but all of the components will keep well if made in advance).

2. When you're ready to serve, divide the rice into bowls. Top with a generous portion of black beans, followed by some pickled onions and a dollop or two of pesto. Finish it off with any additions of your choosing.

3. Leftovers keep well in the refrigerator for up to 5 days. For maximum freshness, store each component separately. When you're ready to serve, gently reheat your desired portions of rice and beans before topping with onions, pesto, and additions.

Prep Time: 15 Minutes

Cook Time: 30 Minutes

Servings: 4

Ingredients

Optional:

- 1 batch crispy baked tofu

Optional:

- 1 ¼ cups brown jasmine rice or long-grain brown rice, rinsed
- 1 tablespoon coconut oil or olive oil
- 1 small white or yellow onion, chopped (about 1 cup)
- Pinch of salt, more to taste
- 1 red bell pepper, sliced into thin (¼" wide) strips
- 1 yellow, orange or green bell pepper, sliced into thin (¼" wide) strips
- 3 carrots, peeled and sliced on the diagonal into ¼" thick rounds (about 1 cup)
- 2 cloves garlic, pressed or minced

- 1 to 2 tablespoons panang curry paste (use 1 for mild or 2 for spicy)
- 1 can (14 ounces) regular coconut milk
- ½ cup water
- 2 tablespoons peanut butter
- 1 tablespoon tamari or soy sauce
- 1 ½ teaspoons coconut sugar or brown sugar
- 2 teaspoons fresh lime juice, to taste

Optional garnishes:

- fresh Thai basil or regular basil, sriracha or chili garlic sauce for extra spice

Instructions

1. If you'd like to serve rice with your curry (optional): Bring a large pot of water to boil. Add the rinsed rice and continue boiling for 30 minutes, reducing heat as necessary to prevent overflow. Remove from heat, drain the rice and return the rice to pot. Cover and let the rice rest for 10 minutes or longer, until you're ready to serve. Just before serving, season the rice to taste with salt and fluff it with a fork.

2. To make the curry, warm a large skillet with deep sides over medium heat. Once it's hot, add the oil. Add the onion and a sprinkle of salt and cook, stirring often, until the onion has softened and is turning translucent, about 5 minutes.

3. Add the bell peppers and carrots. Cook until the bell peppers are easily pierced through by a fork, 3 to 5 more minutes, stirring occasionally. Add the garlic and curry paste and cook, while stirring, for 1 minute.

4. Add the coconut milk and water, and stir to combine. Bring the mixture to a simmer over medium heat. Reduce heat as necessary to maintain a gentle simmer and cook until the peppers and carrots have softened to your liking, about 5 to 10 minutes, stirring occasionally. If you're adding crispy tofu, stir it in now.

5. Remove the pot from the heat. Stir in the peanut butter, tamari, sugar and lime juice. Add salt, to taste (I usually add a pinch or two). If the curry needs a little more punch, add ½ teaspoon more tamari, or for more acidity, add ½ teaspoon more lime juice.

6. Divide rice and curry into bowls and garnish with fresh basil, if using. If you love spicy curries, serve with sriracha or chili garlic sauce on the side.

Prep Time: 10 Minutes

Cook Time: 05 Minutes

Servings: 4

Ingredients

Fig or lemon leaves, for decoration:

- Chunk of good English Cheddar
- Jar of Chutney
- Baked Virginia Ham, thickly sliced, recipe follows
- Crisp apples, cut up
- Celery stalks with leaves, cut in half lengthwise
- Bunch radish, sliced in half
- Soft Hard-Boiled Eggs, recipe follows
- Baby carrots
- Loaf of crusty bread, thickly sliced
- Unsalted butter, softened
- Baked Virginia Ham:
- One 14- to 16-pound fully cooked, spiral-cut smoked ham, on the bone
- 6 garlic cloves

- 8 1/2 ounces mango chutney

- 1/2 cup Dijon mustard

- 1 cup light brown sugar, packed

- 1 orange, zested

- 1/4 cup freshly squeezed orange juice

- Soft Hard-Boiled Eggs:

- 6 extra large eggs

- salt and freshly ground black pepper

Instructions

1. Decoratively arrange the fig or lemon leaves on a serving platter or cutting board. Carefully place the remaining ingredients on top of the leaves and serve.

2. Baked Virginia Ham:

3. Yield: 35 servings for dinner, 50 for cocktails

4. Preheat the oven to 350 degrees F. Place the ham in a heavy roasting pan.

5. Mince the garlic in a food processor fitted with the steel blade. Add the chutney, mustard, brown sugar, orange zest, and orange juice and process until smooth. Pour the glaze over the ham and bake for 1 hour, until the ham is fully heated and the glaze is well browned. Serve hot or at room temperature.

6. 2002, Barefoot Contessa Parties!, All Rights Reserved

Soft Hard-Boiled Eggs:

1. Place the eggs a large saucepan and cover them with cool tap water. Bring the water to a boil, lower the heat and simmer for 3 minutes.
2. Remove the eggs from the saucepan and immediately place them in a bowl of cold water until they are completely cool.
3. Remove the shells, slice each egg in half lengthwise, sprinkle with salt and pepper and serve.

Prep Time: 25 Minutes

Cook Time: 35 Minutes

Servings: 4

Ingredients

- 4 medium cloves garlic, smashed and peeled
- 2 bay leaves
- 1 tablespoon ground cumin
- 1 ¾ teaspoons fine sea salt, divided
- Freshly ground black pepper
- 5 cups water
- 1 cup brown basmati rice (regular, not quick-cooking), rinsed and drained
- 1 cup regular brown or green lentils, picked over for debris, rinsed and drained
- ⅓ cup extra-virgin olive oil
- 2 medium-to-large yellow onions, halved and thinly sliced
- ½ cup thinly sliced green onions (from 1 bunch), divided

- ½ cup chopped fresh cilantro or flat-leaf parsley, divided
- Plain whole-milk or Greek yogurt, for serving
- Spicy sauce, for serving (optional): shatta or zhoug or store-bought chili-garlic sauce or even sriracha

Instructions

1. In a large Dutch oven or soup pot, combine the garlic, bay leaves, cumin, 1 ½ teaspoons of the salt and about 20 twists of freshly ground black pepper. Add the water and bring the mixture to a boil over medium-high heat.

2. Once boiling, stir in the rice and reduce the heat to medium. Cover and cook, stirring occasionally and adjusting the heat as necessary to maintain a controlled simmer, for 10 minutes.

3. Stir in the lentils and let the mixture return to a simmer. Cover again, reduce the heat to medium-low, and cook until the liquid is absorbed and the rice and lentils are tender, about 20 to 23 minutes.

4. Meanwhile, warm the olive oil in a large (12-inch) skillet over medium-high heat. When it's warm enough that a slice of onion sizzles on contact, add the remaining onions. Stir to combine.

5. Stir only every 3 minutes or so at first, then more often once the onions at the edges of the pan start browning. If the onions are browning before they have softened, dial down the heat to give them more time. Cook until the onions are deeply caramelized and starting to crisp at the edges, about 20 to 30 minutes.

In the meantime, line a large plate or cutting board with a couple paper towels.

6. Using a slotted spoon or fish spatula, transfer the onions to the lined plate and spread them evenly across. Sprinkle the remaining ¼ teaspoon salt over the onions. They'll crisp up as they cool.

7. When the lentils and rice are done cooking, drain off any excess water (if there is any) and return the mixture to the pot, off the heat. Lay a kitchen towel across the top of the pot to absorb steam, then cover the pot and let it rest for 10 minutes.

8. Remove the lid, discard the bay leaves, and smash the garlic cloves against the side of the pan with a fork. Add about ¾ths of the green onions and cilantro, reserving the rest for garnish. Gently stir and fluff the rice with a fork. Season to taste with additional salt and pepper, if necessary.

9. Transfer the rice and lentil mixture to a large serving platter or bowl. Top with the caramelized onions and the remaining green onions and cilantro. Serve hot, warm or at room temperature, with yogurt and spicy sauce (optional) on the side.

Prep Time: 30 Minutes

Cook Time: 45 Minutes

Servings: 4

Ingredients

Crispy baked tofu and rice:

- 1 block (12 to 15 ounces) organic extra-firm tofu
- 1 tablespoon extra-virgin olive oil
- 1 tablespoon reduced-sodium tamari or soy sauce
- 1 tablespoon cornstarch or arrowroot starch
- 1 ¼ cups brown basmati rice or long-grain brown rice, rinsed

Peanut sauce:

- ⅓ cup creamy peanut butter
- 3 tablespoons lime juice (about 1 lime)
- 2 tablespoons reduced-sodium tamari or soy sauce
- 1 tablespoon honey or maple syrup, to taste
- 2 teaspoons toasted sesame oil
- 2 garlic cloves, pressed or minced

- ¼ teaspoon red pepper flakes (omit or reduce if sensitive to spice)
- Mango salsa and cabbage
- 2 large ripe mangos, diced
- 1 medium red bell pepper, chopped
- ½ cup (about 4) thinly sliced green onions
- ¼ cup chopped fresh cilantro
- 1 medium jalapeño, seeds and ribs removed, minced
- 2 tablespoons lime juice
- ¼ teaspoon fine sea salt
- 2 cups shredded purple or green cabbage
- Handful of chopped roasted peanuts, for garnish

Instructions

1. Preheat the oven to 400 degrees Fahrenheit and line a large, rimmed baking sheet with parchment paper to prevent the tofu from sticking.

2. To prepare the tofu: Drain the tofu and use your palms to gently squeeze out some of the water. Slice the tofu into thirds lengthwise so you have 3 even slabs. Stack the slabs on top of each other and slice through them lengthwise to make 3 even columns, then slice across to make 5 even rows.

3. Line a cutting board with a lint-free tea towel or paper towels, then arrange the tofu in an even layer on the towel(s). Fold the towel(s) over the cubed tofu, then place something heavy on top (like another cutting board, topped with a cast iron pan or large cans of tomatoes) to help the tofu drain. Let the tofu rest for at least 10 minutes (preferably more like 30 minutes, if you have the time).

4. Meanwhile, bring a large pot of water to boil. Add the rice and boil, uncovered, for 30 minutes. Drain off the remaining cooking water and return the rice to the pot. Cover the pot and let the rice rest, off the heat, for 10 minutes. Fluff with a fork and set aside.

5. Transfer the pressed tofu to the lined baking sheet and drizzle with the olive oil and tamari. Toss to combine. Sprinkle the starch over the tofu, and toss the tofu until the starch is evenly coated, so there are no powdery spots remaining.

6. Arrange the tofu in an even layer. Bake for 25 to 30 minutes, tossing the tofu halfway, until the tofu is deeply golden on the edges. Set aside.

7. Meanwhile, prepare the peanut sauce by whisking all the ingredients together in a bowl. Taste, and if it's too

bold, add another teaspoon of honey to tame it. Set aside.

8. Then, in a medium mixing bowl, combine the diced mango, bell pepper, green onion, cilantro, jalapeño, lime juice and salt. Stir to combine, and set aside.

9. To assemble your bowls, start with a big scoop of cooked rice. Top with a handful (½ cup) shredded cabbage, then a big scoop of mango salsa, a handful of baked tofu, a hefty drizzle of peanut sauce, and a little sprinkle of chopped peanuts. Leftover bowls will keep well in the refrigerator, covered, for about 4 days.

Prep Time: 15 Minutes

Cook Time: 20 Minutes

Servings: 4

Ingredients

- 1 cup uncooked brown basmati rice, for serving (rice is optional, I like to cook extra to have on hand for other meals)
- 2 tablespoons coconut oil or extra-virgin olive oil
- 1 medium yellow onion, chopped
- 1 medium serrano or jalapeño pepper, minced (remove ribs and seeds to tame the spice level)
- ½ teaspoon fine sea salt, to taste
- 5 cloves garlic, pressed or minced (about 1 tablespoon)
- 1 tablespoon peeled and minced fresh ginger (about a 1-inch piece)
- 1 ½ teaspoons garam masala
- 1 ½ teaspoons ground coriander
- ¾ teaspoon ground cumin
- ½ teaspoon ground turmeric

- Pinch of cayenne pepper (optional!)
- 1 large can (28 ounces) fire-roasted crushed tomatoes or whole peeled tomatoes, with their juices
- 2 cans (14 ounces each) chickpeas (or 3 cups cooked chickpeas), rinsed and drained
- Lemon wedges, for garnish
- Fresh cilantro, for garnish (optional)

Instructions

1. Cook the rice (if you want to serve the chana masala on rice): Bring a large pot of water to boil on the stove and rinse the rice in a fine-mesh colander. Once boiling, pour in the rice and give it a stir. Boil the rice for 30 minutes, then turn off the heat and drain the rice. Return the rice to the pot and cover the pot. Let the rice steam for 10 minutes. Remove the lid, fluff the rice with a fork and season with sea salt to taste.

2. Cook the chana masala: In a medium Dutch oven or large saucepan, warm the oil over medium-low heat. Add the onion, serrano and salt. Cook until the onion is tender and turning translucent, about 5 minutes.

3. Add the garlic and ginger, and cook until fragrant, about 30 seconds to 1 minute. Stir in the garam

masala, coriander, cumin, turmeric, salt and cayenne (if using), and cook for another minute, while stirring constantly.

4. Add the tomatoes and their juices. If using whole tomatoes, use the back of a wooden spoon to break the tomatoes apart (you can leave some chunks of tomato for texture).

5. Raise the heat to medium-high and add the chickpeas. Bring the mixture to a simmer. Cook, reducing the heat as necessary to maintain a gentle simmer, for 10 minutes or longer to allow the flavors to develop. Season to taste with additional salt, if desired. If it's not spicy enough for your liking, add another pinch of cayenne.

6. Serve over basmati rice, if desired, and garnish with a lemon wedge or two and a sprinkle of fresh cilantro leaves.

Prep Time: 35 Minutes

Cook Time: 30 Minutes

Servings: 9

Ingredients

Cashew cream:

- 2 cups raw cashews, soaked for at least 4 hours if you do not have a high-powered blender
- 1 cup water
- 2 tablespoons lemon juice
- 2 teaspoons apple cider vinegar
- ¾ teaspoon fine sea salt
- ½ teaspoon Dijon mustard

Vegetables:

- 2 tablespoons extra-virgin olive oil
- 1 medium-to-large yellow onion, chopped
- 2 large or 3 medium carrots, chopped (about 1 cup)
- 8 ounces Baby Bella mushrooms, cleaned and chopped
- ½ teaspoon fine sea salt, to taste

- Freshly ground black pepper, to taste
- 5 to 6 ounces baby spinach, roughly chopped
- 2 cloves garlic, pressed or minced

Everything else:

- 2 ½ cups marinara sauce, homemade or store-bought
- 9 no-boil lasagna noodles
- Suggested garnishes: vegan Parmesan (or a light sprinkle of nutritional yeast) and fresh basil

Instructions

1. Preheat the oven to 425 degrees Fahrenheit. If you soaked your cashews, drain and rinse them until the water runs clear.
2. In a blender, combine the cashews, water, lemon juice, vinegar, salt, and mustard. Blend until the mixture is smooth and creamy, stopping to scrape down the sides as necessary. If you're having trouble blending the mixture, slowly blend in up to ½ cup additional water, using only as much as necessary. Set aside.
3. Then, we'll prepare the vegetables: In a large skillet over medium heat, warm the olive oil. Once

shimmering, add the onion, carrots, mushrooms, salt and several twists of black pepper. Cook, stirring every couple of minutes, until most of the moisture is gone and the vegetables are tender and turning golden on the edges, about 8 to 10 minutes. Add another splash of olive oil if necessary to prevent them from sticking to the bottom of the pan.

4. Add a few large handfuls of spinach to the skillet. Cook, stirring frequently, until the spinach has wilted. Repeat with remaining spinach and cook until all of the spinach has wilted, about 3 minutes. Add the garlic and cook until fragrant, stirring constantly, about 30 seconds. Remove the skillet from the heat and season to taste with salt and pepper.

5. Spread ¾ cup tomato sauce evenly over the bottom of a 9" by 9" baking dish. Layer 3 lasagna noodles on top (snap off their ends to fit, and/or overlap their edges as necessary). Spread 1 cup of the cashew cream evenly over the noodles. Top with half of the veggies. Top with ¾ cup tomato sauce.

6. Top with 3 more noodles, followed by another 1 cup cashew cream (save the leftover cream). Then add the remaining veggies.

7. Top with 3 more noodles, then spread ¾ cup tomato sauce over the top to evenly cover the noodles.

8. Wrap a sheet of parchment paper or aluminum foil around the top of the lasagna, making sure it's taut so it doesn't touch the top. Bake, covered, for 25 minutes, then remove the cover, rotate the pan by 180° and continue cooking for about 5 to 10 more minutes, until it's steaming and lightly bubbling at the corners.

9. Remove the pan from the oven and let the lasagna cool for 15 to 20 minutes, so it has time to set and cool down to a reasonable temperature. Drizzle leftover cashew cream on top (if it's too thick to drizzle, thin it out with a small amount of water first). Sprinkle vegan Parmesan and fresh basil on top, if using, then slice and serve.

21. Italian Eggplant Parmesan

Prep Time: 15 Minutes

Cook Time: 45 Minutes

Servings: 6-9

Ingredients

- 3 pounds eggplants (about 3 smallish or 2 medium)
- ¼ cup + 2 tablespoons extra-virgin olive oil, divided
- Fine sea salt and freshly ground black pepper
- 1 medium yellow onion, finely chopped
- 2 cloves garlic, pressed or minced
- ¼ cup tomato paste
- 28 ounces crushed tomatoes, preferably the fire-roasted variety
- ¼ cup roughly chopped fresh basil, plus additional basil for garnish
- 1 teaspoon balsamic vinegar
- Pinch of red pepper flakes
- 6 ounces freshly grated part-skim mozzarella cheese (about 1 ½ cups, packed)

- 2 ounces freshly grated Parmesan cheese (about 1 cup)

Instructions

1. To roast the eggplant: Preheat the oven to 425 degrees Fahrenheit with racks in the lower and upper thirds of the oven. Line two large rimmed, baking sheets with parchment paper for easy cleanup.

2. Slice off both rounded ends on one eggplant, then stand it up on its widest flat side. Slice through the eggplant vertically to make long, even slabs ¼- to ½-inch-thick. Discard both of the sides that are covered in eggplant skin. Repeat with the other eggplant(s).

3. Brush both sides of the eggplant slabs lightly with olive oil (you'll likely need about ¼ cup oil). Arrange them in a single layer on the prepared baking sheets. Sprinkle the top sides with a few dashes of salt and pepper. Roast until golden and tender, about 22 to 27 minutes—halfway through baking, rotate the pans 180 degrees and swap their positions (move pan on lower rack to upper rack, and vice versa). The pan on the lower rack might need a few extra minutes in the oven to turn golden. Set aside.

4. Meanwhile, to make the tomato sauce: In a medium saucepan over medium heat, warm 2 tablespoons olive oil until shimmering. Add the onion and a pinch of salt. Cook, stirring occasionally, until the onion is very tender and translucent, about 4 to 7 minutes.

5. Add the garlic and tomato paste. Cook, while stirring, about 1 minute. Add the crushed tomatoes, stir to combine, and bring the mixture to a simmer. Once simmering, reduce the heat to medium-low and simmer until the sauce has thickened nicely, about 15 minutes. Remove the pot from the heat and stir in the chopped basil, vinegar, salt and red pepper flakes. Taste, and add more salt if necessary (I usually add another ¼ teaspoon).

6. When you're ready to assemble, spread about ¾ cup of the sauce in the bottom of a 9" square baker. Arrange about one-third of the eggplant slices over the sauce, overlapping slightly (cut them to fit, if necessary). Spoon another ¾ cup of the sauce over the eggplant and sprinkle with ¼ cup mozzarella cheese.

7. Arrange about half of the remaining eggplant slices evenly on top. Spread another ¾ cup sauce on top and sprinkle with ¼ cup mozzarella cheese. Layer the

remaining eggplant slices on top and top with ¾ cup sauce (you might have a little left over) and the remaining mozzarella cheese. Evenly sprinkle the Parmesan on top.

8. Bake on the lower rack at 425 degrees Fahrenheit, uncovered, until the sauce bubbles and the top is golden, about 20 to 25 minutes. Let it cool for at least 15 minutes to give it time to set, then chop and sprinkle additional basil on top. Slice with a sharp knife and serve.

9. Leftovers keep well, covered and refrigerated, for about 4 days. Reheat before serving.

Prep Time: 15 Minutes

Cook Time: 60 Minutes

Servings: 6-9

Ingredients

- 3 tablespoons extra-virgin olive oil, divided
- 1 medium yellow onion, chopped fine
- 1 ½ teaspoons fine sea salt, divided
- 6 garlic cloves, pressed or minced
- 2 teaspoons smoked paprika
- 1 can (15 ounces) diced tomatoes (preferably the fire-roasted variety), drained
- 2 cups short-grain brown rice
- 1 can (15 ounces) chickpeas, rinsed and drained, or 1 ½ cups cooked chickpeas
- 3 cups vegetable broth
- ⅓ cup dry white wine or vegetable broth
- ½ teaspoon saffron threads, crumbled (optional)
- 1 can (14 ounces) quartered artichokes or 1 jar (12 ounces) marinated artichoke, drained

- 2 red bell peppers, stemmed, seeded and sliced into long, ½"-wide strips
- ½ cup Kalamata olives, pitted and halved
- Freshly ground black pepper
- ¼ cup chopped fresh parsley, plus about 1 tablespoon more for garnish
- 2 tablespoons lemon juice, plus additional lemon wedges for garnish
- ½ cup frozen peas

Instructions

1. Arrange your oven racks in the upper and lower thirds of the oven, making sure that you have ample space between the two racks for your Dutch oven. You're going to need a large Dutch oven (preferably 6 quarts/11-to-12" in diameter or bigger, although I got by with my 5.5-quart Le Creuset) or a large skillet with a snug-fitting lid (both must be oven-safe!).

2. Preheat the oven to 350 degrees Fahrenheit. Heat 2 tablespoons of the oil in your Dutch oven or skillet over medium heat until shimmering. Add the onion and a pinch of salt. Cook until the onions are tender and translucent, about 5 minutes.

3. Stir in the garlic and paprika and cook until fragrant, about 30 seconds. Stir in the tomatoes and cook until the mixture begins to darken and thicken slightly, about 2 minutes Stir in the rice and cook until the grains are well coated with tomato mixture, about 1 minute. Stir in the chickpeas, broth, wine, saffron (if using) and 1 teaspoon salt.

4. Increase the heat to medium-high and bring the mixture to a boil, stirring occasionally. Cover the pot and transfer it to the lower rack in the oven. Bake, undisturbed, until the liquid is absorbed and the rice is tender, 50 to 55 minutes.

5. Meanwhile, line a large, rimmed baking sheet with parchment paper for easy cleanup. On the baking sheet, combine the artichoke, peppers, chopped olives, 1 tablespoon of the olive oil, ½ teaspoon of the salt, and about 10 twists of freshly ground black pepper. Toss to combine, then spread the contents evenly across the pan.

6. Roast the vegetables on the upper rack until the artichokes and peppers are tender and browned around the edges, about 40 to 45 minutes. Remove from the oven and let the vegetables cool for a few minutes. Add ¼ cup parsley to the pan and the lemon

juice, and toss to combine. Season with salt and pepper, to taste. Set aside.

7. For optional socarrat (crispy bottom—beware that you might have to scrub burnt bits from your pot later if you do this): Uncover the pot of baked rice, transfer it to the stovetop and cook over medium-high heat for about 5 minutes, rotating the pot as needed, until the bottom layer of rice is well browned and crisp.

8. Socarrat or not, sprinkle the peas and roasted vegetables over the baked rice, cover, and let the paella sit for 5 minutes. Garnish with a sprinkle of chopped parsley (about 1 tablespoon) and serve in individual bowls, with lemon wedges on the side.

Prep Time: 30 Minutes

Cook Time: 30 Minutes

Servings: 4

Ingredients

- 2 tablespoons vegetable oil
- 2 cloves garlic, finely grated with a rasp
- 1 tablespoon fresh ginger, grated with a rasp
- 3 scallions, thinly sliced, greens and whites separated
- 4 ounces shiitake mushrooms, sliced
- 5 cups chicken bone broth or low-sodium chicken broth
- 4 heads baby bok choy, quartered lengthwise
- 2 tablespoons soy sauce
- One 12-ounce package frozen wontons (about 20)
- Salt

Instructions

1. In a medium pot or Dutch oven, heat the vegetable oil over medium heat. Add the garlic, ginger and white

parts of the scallions and cook, stirring frequently, until fragrant, 1 to 2 minutes. Add the shiitakes and cook until they begin to soften, another minute.

2. Add the bone broth and bring to a boil. Add the bok choy and simmer, stirring occasionally, until the bok choy is tender, 4 to 5 minutes. Add the soy sauce and stir. Add the wontons and cook until they are cooked through, 2 to 3 minutes. Taste and season if necessary.

3. Ladle into bowls, then top with the scallion greens. Serve immediately.

Prep Time: 20 Minutes

Cook Time: 55 Minutes

Servings: 6-8

Ingredients

- 1 tablespoon canola oil
- Two 10-ounce cans diced tomatoes with chiles, such as Rotel
- 1 cup chicken broth
- 1 tablespoon chili powder
- 1 teaspoon ground cumin
- 1/2 teaspoon salt
- One 15.5-ounce can black beans, drained and rinsed
- One 10-ounce bag frozen corn
- 5 cups shredded cooked chicken (from about 1 small rotisserie chicken)
- 12 small corn tortillas, cut into quarters
- One 8-ounce block Monterey Jack cheese, shredded (about 2 cups)
- 1/2 cup sour cream
- 1/3 cup diced red onion

- 1/3 cup loosely packed fresh cilantro, chopped

Instructions

1. Preheat the oven to 375 degrees F. Brush a 9-by-13-inch casserole dish with the oil.

2. Stir together the diced tomatoes with chiles, chicken broth, chili powder, cumin and salt in a large bowl. Add the black beans, frozen corn, chicken, tortilla wedges and half the cheese and stir to evenly distribute and moisten all of the ingredients. Transfer to the prepared casserole dish and spread into an even layer. Loosely cover with aluminum foil and bake for 25 minutes.

3. Raise the oven temperature to 400 degrees F. Remove the foil and sprinkle the top with the remaining cheese. Continue to bake until the cheese is melted and just starting to brown, about 10 minutes. Top with dollops of sour cream and sprinkle with the red onion and cilantro. Serve hot.

Prep Time: 20 Minutes

Cook Time: 55 Minutes

Servings: 4-6

Ingredients

- Nonstick cooking spray
- 2 cups low-sodium vegetable broth
- One 13.5-ounce can unsweetened coconut milk
- 4 cloves garlic, finely grated
- 1 tablespoon finely grated peeled fresh ginger (from a 1- to 2-inch piece)
- 1 serrano chile pepper, stemmed and finely chopped (remove seeds for less heat)
- 2 1/2 teaspoons curry powder, preferably Madras
- Salt
- Two 15.5-ounce cans chickpeas, drained and rinsed
- 2 cups lightly packed baby spinach, roughly chopped
- 1 1/2 cups basmati rice
- 1/2 medium head cauliflower, cut into small florets (about 3 heaping cups)
- 1/2 small red onion, thinly sliced

- Cilantro leaves, plain whole-milk yogurt and lime wedges, for serving

Instructions

1. Preheat the oven to 425 degrees F. Spray a 9-by-13-inch baking dish with nonstick spray.

2. Whisk the vegetable broth, coconut milk, garlic, ginger, serrano, curry powder and 2 teaspoons salt together in a medium bowl until combined. Add the chickpeas and spinach and stir to coat.

3. Spread the rice evenly in the bottom of the prepared dish. Pour in the coconut-milk mixture, distributing the chickpeas and spinach evenly over the rice. Scatter the cauliflower and onion over the top, making sure to go all the way to the edge of the pan (it's okay if the cauliflower is not completely submerged in liquid).

4. Cover tightly with foil and bake until the vegetables have softened but are still vibrant, about 25 minutes. Remove the foil and bake until the cauliflower is charred in spots and the rice is cooked through, 20 to 25 minutes more. Let sit for 5 minutes to allow the rice to absorb more of the moisture. Serve topped with

cilantro, a drizzle of yogurt and lime wedges for squeezing.

Prep Time: 30 Minutes

Cook Time: 1hrs 20 Minutes

Servings: 12-16

Ingredients

- 8 baking potatoes, washed
- 3 tablespoons canola oil
- 2 sticks salted butter
- 1 cup bacon bits (fry your own!)
- 1 cup sour cream
- 1 cup Cheddar or Jack cheese (or a mix of both), plus more for topping
- 1 cup whole milk
- 2 teaspoons seasoned salt
- 3 green onions, sliced
- Freshly ground black pepper

Instructions

1. Preheat the oven to 400 degrees F.

2. Place the potatoes on a baking sheet. Rub them with the canola oil and bake for 1 hour, making sure they're sufficiently cooked through.

3. Slice the butter into pats. Place in a large mixing bowl and add the bacon bits and sour cream. Remove the potatoes from the oven. Lower the heat to 350 degrees F.

4. With a sharp knife, cut each potato in half lengthwise. Scrape out the insides into the mixing bowl, being careful not to tear the shell. Leave a small rim of potato intact for support. Lay the hollowed out potato shells on a baking sheet.

5. Smash the potatoes into the butter, bacon and sour cream. Add the cheese, milk, seasoned salt, green onions and black pepper to taste and mix together well. (IMPORTANT: If you plan to freeze the twice-baked potatoes, do NOT add the green onions.)

6. Fill the potato shells with the filling. I like to fill the shells so they look abundant and heaping. Top each potato with a little more grated cheese and pop 'em in the oven until the potato is warmed through, 15 to 20 minutes.

Prep Time: 20 Minutes

Cook Time: 1hrs 20 Minutes

Servings: 12

Ingredients

- 1/4 cup good olive oil
- 1 cup chopped yellow onion
- 3 scallions, white and green parts, chopped
- 2 (10-ounce) packages frozen chopped spinach, defrosted
- 4 extra-large eggs, lightly beaten
- 3 tablespoons freshly grated Parmesan cheese
- Plain dry bread crumbs
- 1 teaspoon grated nutmeg
- 2 teaspoons salt
- 1 teaspoon freshly ground black pepper
- 2 cups small-diced feta cheese (12 ounces)
- 3 tablespoons toasted pine nuts
- 24 sheets frozen phyllo dough, defrosted
- 1/4 pound (1 stick) unsalted butter, melted
- Flaked sea salt, such as Maldon, for sprinkling

Instructions

1. Preheat the oven to 375 degrees F.

2. Heat the olive oil in a medium saute pan, add the onion, and cook for 5 minutes over medium-low heat. Add the scallions, and cook for another 2 minutes until the scallions are wilted but still green. Meanwhile, gently squeeze most of the water out of the spinach and place it in a large bowl.

3. When the onion and scallions are done, add them to the spinach. Mix in the eggs, Parmesan cheese, 3 tablespoons bread crumbs, the nutmeg, salt, and pepper. Gently fold in the feta and pine nuts.

4. Place 1 sheet of phyllo dough flat on a work surface with the long end in front of you. Brush the dough lightly with butter and sprinkle it with a teaspoon of bread crumbs. Working quickly, slide another sheet of phyllo dough on top of the first, brush it with butter, and sprinkle lightly with bread crumbs. (Use just enough bread crumbs so the layers of phyllo don't stick together.) Pile 4 layers total on top of each other this way, brushing each with butter and sprinkling with bread crumbs. Cut the sheets of phyllo in half lengthwise. Place 1/3 cup spinach filling on the shorter end and roll the phyllo up diagonally as if

folding a flag. Then fold the triangle of phyllo over straight and then diagonally again. Continue folding first diagonally and then straight until you reach the end of the sheet. The filling should be totally enclosed. Continue assembling phyllo layers and folding the filling until all of the filling is used. Place on a sheet pan, seam sides down. Brush with melted butter, sprinkle with flaked salt, and bake for 30 to 35 minutes, until the phyllo is browned and crisp. Serve hot.

Prep Time: 30 Minutes

Cook Time: 1hrs 30 Minutes

Servings: 8

Ingredients

- 1 (5 to 6 pound) roasting chicken
- salt
- Freshly ground black pepper
- 1 large bunch fresh thyme, plus 20 sprigs
- 1 lemon, halved
- 1 head garlic, cut in half crosswise
- 2 tablespoons (1/4 stick) butter, melted
- 1 large yellow onion, thickly sliced
- 4 carrots cut into 2-inch chunks
- 1 bulb of fennel, tops removed, and cut into wedges
- Olive oil

Instructions

1. Preheat the oven to 425 degrees F.

2. Remove the chicken giblets. Rinse the chicken inside and out. Remove any excess fat and leftover pin feathers and pat the outside dry. Liberally salt and pepper the inside of the chicken. Stuff the cavity with the bunch of thyme, both halves of lemon, and all the garlic. Brush the outside of the chicken with the butter and sprinkle again with salt and pepper. Tie the legs together with kitchen string and tuck the wing tips under the body of the chicken. Place the onions, carrots, and fennel in a roasting pan. Toss with salt, pepper, 20 sprigs of thyme, and olive oil. Spread around the bottom of the roasting pan and place the chicken on top.

3. Roast the chicken for 1 1/2 hours, or until the juices run clear when you cut between a leg and thigh. Remove the chicken and vegetables to a platter and cover with aluminum foil for about 20 minutes. Slice the chicken onto a platter and serve it with the vegetables.

Prep Time: 20 Minutes

Cook Time: 30 Minutes

Servings: 4

Ingredients

- 4 (1/2-inch thick) slices sandwich bread
- 2 teaspoons melted unsalted butter, plus 6 tablespoons cold unsalted butter, cut into pieces
- 4 (1/8-inch thick) slices boiled ham
- 4 (6 to 7-ounce) boneless, skinless chicken breast halves
- 1 teaspoon Essence or Creole Seasoning, recipe follows
- 1/2 teaspoon salt, plus more for seasoning chicken
- 1/4 teaspoon freshly ground black pepper, plus more for seasoning chicken
- 1 tablespoon olive oil
- 1/4 cup minced shallots
- 2 teaspoons minced garlic
- 1/2 teaspoon herbes de Provence
- 1 tablespoon tomato paste

- 1/2 cup dry white wine

- 2 cups peeled, seededand chopped fresh tomatoes

- 1 1/2 cups chicken stock or canned low-sodium chicken broth

- 1/2 cup heavy cream

- Chopped fresh parsley leaves, for garnish

- Emeril's ESSENCE Creole Seasoning (also referred to as Bayou Blast):

- 2 1/2 tablespoons paprika

- 2 tablespoons salt2 tablespoons garlic powder

- 1 tablespoon black pepper

- 1 tablespoon onion powder

- 1 tablespoon cayenne pepper

- 1 tablespoon dried oregano

- 1 tablespoon dried thyme

Instructions

1. Preheat the oven to 400 degrees F. Line a small baking sheet with aluminum foil and set aside.

2. Toast the bread until light golden brown on both sides. Trim the toast using a 4-inch round cookie cutter and using a pastry brush, lightly coat 1 side of each toast with 1/2 teaspoon of the melted butter. Set

aside on a wire rack to crisp. Reserve trimmed crusts and crumble into coarse bread crumbs to be used as garnish.

3. In a large nonstick skillet or saute pan sear the ham slices until lightly golden, about 1 minute.

4. Set aside.

5. Season each chicken breast with 1/4 teaspoon of the Essence and season lightly with salt and pepper.

6. In the already hot large skillet or saute pan, heat the oil over high heat. Add the chicken and sear until lightly colored, about 1 1/2 minutes per side. Transfer the chicken to the prepared baking sheet and cook until cooked through, 12 to 14 minutes.

7. While the chicken breasts are finishing in the oven, make the pan sauce: Return the skillet to medium-high heat and melt 2 tablespoons of the butter in the fat and juices remaining in the pan. When the butter is foamy, add the shallots, salt, and pepper and cook, stirring, until the shallots are soft, about 2 minutes. Add the garlic and herbes de Provence and cook, stirring, for 30 seconds. Add the tomato paste, wine, and tomatoes; bring to a boil, and cook, stirring, until the wine is reduced, about 1 minute. Add the stock,

return to the boil, and cook until the mixture is reduced by half, about 8 minutes.

8. Add the heavy cream, stir, and place the chicken breasts in the pan. Top each chicken breast with a piece of ham and baste with the sauce; continue to cook until sauce is thick enough to coat the back of a spoon, about 5 minutes. Reduce the heat to low and swirl in the remaining 4 tablespoons butter, a piece or 2 at a time. Remove from the heat, adjust the seasoning to taste, and cover to keep warm until ready to serve.

9. To serve, place 1 toast round in the center of 4 large plates and place 1 ham-topped chicken breast on top. Drizzle each portion with the sauce, garnish with chopped fresh parsley and the reserved bread crumbs and serve immediately.

Prep Time: 20 Minutes

Cook Time: 30 Minutes

Servings: 4

Ingredients

- 1 pound Yukon gold potatoes, cut into -inch cubes
- salt
- 3 scallions, chopped
- 4 turkey cutlets (about 1 pound)
- 1 1/2 teaspoons smoked paprika
- Freshly ground pepper
- 2 tablespoons vegetable oil
- 1 cup low-sodium chicken broth
- 1 tablespoon dijon mustard
- 4 tablespoons cold unsalted butter, diced
- 2 cups frozen peas (about 10 ounces), thawed
- 1 lemon (half zested, half cut into wedges)
- 2 tablespoons chopped fresh parsley

Instructions

1. Put the potatoes in a pot and cover with water by 1 inch; season with salt. Bring to a boil. Reduce the heat to medium and simmer until tender, about 8 minutes, adding the scallions during the last minute. Drain.

2. Meanwhile, season the turkey with the paprika, 1/2 teaspoon salt and a few grinds of pepper. Heat the vegetable oil in a large skillet over medium heat. Add the turkey and cook until browned and cooked through, about 3 minutes per side; remove to a plate.

3. Add the broth to the skillet, scraping the pan with a wooden spoon. Cook until reduced by half, about 5 minutes. Stir in the mustard and half of the butter. Season with salt and pepper; set aside.

4. Melt the remaining butter in the pot used for the potatoes over medium heat. Add the potatoes, 1/4 cup water, the peas, lemon zest, parsley and a pinch each of salt and pepper. Cook until the peas are tender, 3 minutes. Serve with the turkey, pan sauce and lemon wedges.